Table of Contents

Introduction

Parkinson's disease (PD), or simply Parkinson's is a long-term degenerative disorder of the central nervous system that mainly affects the motor system. The symptoms usually emerge slowly and, as the disease worsens, non-motor symptoms become more common. The most obvious early symptoms are tremor, rigidity, slowness of movement, and difficulty with walking, but cognitive and behavioral problems may also occur. Parkinson's disease dementia becomes common in the advanced stages of the disease. Depression and anxiety are also common, occurring in more than a third of people with PD. Other symptoms include sensory, sleep, and emotional problems. The main motor symptoms are collectively called "parkinsonism", or a "parkinsonian syndrome"

Parkinson's disease is a brain disorder that leads to shaking, stiffness, and difficulty with walking, balance, and coordination.Older woman and her caregiver Parkinson's symptoms usually begin gradually and get worse over time. As the disease progresses, people may have difficulty walking and talking. They may also have mental and behavioral changes, sleep problems, depression, memory difficulties, and fatigue.

Both men and women can have Parkinson's disease. However, the disease affects about 50 percent more men than women.

One clear risk factor for Parkinson's is age. Although most people with Parkinson's first develop the disease at about age 60, about 5 to 10 percent of people with Parkinson's have "early-onset" disease, which begins before the age of 50. Early-onset forms of Parkinson's are often, but not always, inherited, and some forms have been linked to specific gene mutations.

What Causes Parkinson's Disease?

Parkinson's disease occurs when nerve cells, or neurons, in an area of the brain that controls movement become impaired and/or die. Normally, these neurons produce an important brain chemical known as dopamine. When the neurons die or become impaired, they produce less dopamine, which causes the movement problems of Parkinson's. Scientists still do not know what causes cells that produce dopamine to die.

People with Parkinson's also lose the nerve endings that produce norepinephrine, the main chemical messenger of the sympathetic nervous system, which controls many automatic functions of the body, such as heart rate and blood pressure. The loss of norepinephrine might help explain some of the non-movement features of Parkinson's, such as fatigue, irregular blood pressure, decreased movement of food through the digestive tract, and sudden drop in blood pressure when a person stands up from a sitting or lying-down position.

Many brain cells of people with Parkinson's contain Lewy bodies, unusual clumps of the protein alpha-synuclein. Scientists are trying to better understand the normal and abnormal functions of alpha-synuclein and its relationship to genetic mutations that impact Parkinson's disease and Lewy body dementia.

Although some cases of Parkinson's appear to be hereditary, and a few can be traced to specific genetic mutations, in most cases the disease occurs randomly and does not seem to run in families. Many researchers now believe that Parkinson's disease results from a combination of genetic factors and environmental factors such as exposure to toxins.

Early signs

Here are some early signs of Parkinson's disease:

- Movement: There may be a tremor in the hands.
- Coordination: A reduced sense of coordination and balance can cause people to drop items they are holding. They may be more likely to fall.
- Gait: The person's posture may change, so that they lean forward slightly, as if they were hurrying. They may also develop a shuffling gait.
- Facial expression: This can become fixed, due to changes in the nerves that control facial muscles.
- Voice: There may be a tremor in the voice, or the person may speak more softly than before.
- Handwriting: This may become more cramped and smaller.
- Sense of smell: A loss of sense of smell can be an early sign.

- Sleep problems: These are a feature of Parkinson's, and they may be an early sign. Restless legs may contribute to this.

Other common symptoms include:

- mood changes, including depression
- difficulty chewing and swallowing
- problems with urination
- constipation
- skin problems
- sleep problems
- REM sleep disorder: Authors of a study published in 2015 describe another neurological condition, REM sleep disorder, as a "powerful predictor" for Parkinson's disease and some other neurological conditions.

The Importance Of Recognizing Early Symptoms

Many people think that the early signs of Parkinson's are normal signs of aging. For this reason, they may not seek help.

However, treatment is more likely to be effective if a person takes it early in the development of Parkinson's disease. For this reason, it is important to get an early diagnosis if possible. If treatment does not start until the person has clear symptoms, it will not be as effective.

Moreover, a number of other conditions can have similar symptoms.

These include

- drug-induced Parkinsonism
- head trauma
- encephalitis
- stroke
- Lewy body dementia
- corticobasal degeneration
- multiple system atrophy
- progressive supranuclear palsy

The similarity to other conditions can make it hard for doctors to diagnose Parkinson's disease in the early stages.

Movement symptoms may start on one side of the body and gradually affect both sides.

Complications

Parkinson's disease is often accompanied by these additional problems, which may be treatable:

- Thinking difficulties. You may experience cognitive problems (dementia) and thinking difficulties. These usually occur in the later stages of Parkinson's disease. Such cognitive problems aren't very responsive to medications.

- Depression and emotional changes. You may experience depression, sometimes in the very early stages. Receiving treatment for depression can make it easier to handle the other challenges of Parkinson's disease.

- You may also experience other emotional changes, such as fear, anxiety or loss of motivation. Doctors may give you medications to treat these symptoms.

- Swallowing problems. You may develop difficulties with swallowing as your condition progresses. Saliva may accumulate in your mouth due to slowed swallowing, leading to drooling.

- Chewing and eating problems. Late-stage Parkinson's disease affects the muscles in your mouth, making chewing difficult. This can lead to choking and poor nutrition.

- Sleep problems and sleep disorders. People with Parkinson's disease often have sleep problems, including waking up frequently throughout the night, waking up early or falling asleep during the day.

- People may also experience rapid eye movement sleep behavior disorder, which involves acting out your dreams. Medications may help your sleep problems.

- Bladder problems. Parkinson's disease may cause bladder problems, including being unable to control urine or having difficulty urinating.

- Constipation. Many people with Parkinson's disease develop constipation, mainly due to a slower digestive tract.

You may also experience:

- Blood pressure changes. You may feel dizzy or lightheaded when you stand due to a sudden drop in blood pressure (orthostatic hypotension).
- Smell dysfunction. You may experience problems with your sense of smell. You may have difficulty identifying certain odors or the difference between odors.
- Fatigue. Many people with Parkinson's disease lose energy and experience fatigue, especially later in the day. The cause isn't always known.
- Pain. Some people with Parkinson's disease experience pain, either in specific areas of their bodies or throughout their bodies.
- Sexual dysfunction. Some people with Parkinson's disease notice a decrease in sexual desire or performance.

Diagnosis of Parkinson's Disease

A number of disorders can cause symptoms similar to those of Parkinson's disease. People with Parkinson's-like symptoms that result from other causes are sometimes said to have parkinsonism. While these disorders initially may be misdiagnosed as Parkinson's, certain medical tests, as well as response to drug treatment, may help to distinguish them from Parkinson's. Since many other diseases have similar features but require different treatments, it is important to make an exact diagnosis as soon as possible.

There are currently no blood or laboratory tests to diagnose nongenetic cases of Parkinson's disease. Diagnosis is based on a person's medical history and a neurological examination. Improvement after initiating medication is another important hallmark of Parkinson's disease.

Treatment of Parkinson's Disease

Although there is no cure for Parkinson's disease, medicines, surgical treatment, and other therapies can often relieve some symptoms.

Medicines for Parkinson's Disease

Medicines prescribed for Parkinson's include:

Drugs that increase the level of dopamine in the brain

Drugs that affect other brain chemicals in the body

Drugs that help control nonmotor symptoms

The main therapy for Parkinson's is levodopa, also called L-dopa. Nerve cells use levodopa to make dopamine to replenish the brain's dwindling supply. Usually, people take levodopa along with another medication called carbidopa. Carbidopa prevents or reduces some of the side effects of levodopa therapy—such as nausea, vomiting, low blood pressure, and restlessness—and reduces the amount of levodopa needed to improve symptoms.

People with Parkinson's should never stop taking levodopa without telling their doctor. Suddenly stopping the drug may have serious side effects, such as being unable to move or having difficulty breathing.

Other medicines used to treat Parkinson's symptoms include:

Dopamine agonists to mimic the role of dopamine in the brain

MAO-B inhibitors to slow down an enzyme that breaks down dopamine in the brain

COMT inhibitors to help break down dopamine

Amantadine, an old antiviral drug, to reduce involuntary movements

Anticholinergic drugs to reduce tremors and muscle rigidity

Deep Brain Stimulation

For people with Parkinson's who do not respond well to medications, deep brain stimulation, or DBS, may be appropriate. DBS is a surgical procedure that surgically implants electrodes into part of the brain and connects them to a small electrical device implanted in the chest. The device and electrodes painlessly stimulate the brain in a way that helps stop many of the movement-related symptoms of Parkinson's, such as tremor, slowness of movement, and rigidity.

Determining Candidates for DBS

In deciding candidates for DBS, a good carbidopa/levodopa (Sinamet) profile is considered a key determinant for success. A person with a good Sinamet profile:

Shows dramatic improvement in response to Sinamet

Experiences a dramatic difference between "on" and "off" states

Appears near normal in the "on" state

Spends most of the day "off"

Deep brain stimulation has shown good results with certain symptoms of PD while having little effect on other common symptoms. Dyskinesias and tremor are the symptoms most commonly helped. DBS can reduce on/off fluctuations (more "on" and less "off") and can also address:

Dyskinesias

Tremor

Stiffness

Slowness of movement, including freezing episodes

Shuffling gait

Deep brain stimulation does not help:

Swallowing problems

Softness of speech

Constipation

Drooling

Memory difficulties

Other Therapies

Other therapies may be used to help with Parkinson's disease symptoms. They include physical, occupational, and speech therapies, which help with gait and voice disorders, tremors and rigidity, and decline in mental functions. Other supportive therapies include a healthy diet and exercises to strengthen muscles and improve balance.

Medical Management of Parkinson's Disease

Because diagnosis is based on medical history, neurologic examination, and observation over time, a correct diagnosis is critical for effective management of the disease. Since many other diseases have similar features (especially when symptoms are mild), a timely and precise diagnosis is important so that patients can receive the proper and early treatment.

Brain scans and laboratory tests can be used to rule out other diseases but commuted tomography (CT) and magnetic resonance imaging (MRI) brain scans of people with PD usually appear normal. Cellular changes that occur on a microscopic, chemical level cannot be reliably detected by scans or blood tests.

Although there is progress on tests that can identify the presence of PD in vivo, Parkinson's can currently only be definitively confirmed through its pathologic hallmark of Lewy bodies and Lewy neurites upon postmortem analysis (Haas et al., 2012). In the absence of confirming tests, the patient's response to levodopa is often used to confirm the presence of PD.

There is a consensus among clinicians and researchers that new medical treatments for Parkinson's disease should move from treating symptoms to modifying the disease pathology. The ultimate goal is to find neuroprotective treatments that stop or even prevent neurologic degeneration.

Symptomatic Treatment

Symptomatic Parkinson's disease therapies are designed to alleviate motor and nonmotor symptoms, delay the progression of the disease, and manage the side effects of treatment. The challenge faced by clinicians is to find best treatments for each patient, re-evaluating as symptoms change. Among the many symptoms that occur in PD, cognitive changes, fatigue, anxiety and depression, sleep disturbances, and bladder and bowel dysfunction are usually treated successfully with a variety of drugs.

Early PD symptoms can be vague: increased clumsiness with the hands, mild gait irregularities, and intermittent tremor that is most obvious when the hand is resting or suspended when walking. Tremor, when present, is regular and rhythmic. A number of nonmotor symptoms such as loss of smell, sleep disturbances, sensory changes, and pain can occur well before motor symptoms are evident.

Dopamine Replacement

The pharmacologic mainstay for the treatment of Parkinson's disease is the replacement of dopamine with levodopa, a precursor of dopamine. Dopamine replacement poses many challenges because only about 10% of a levodopa dose actually crosses the blood–brain barrier and enters the brain. The remaining levodopa is susceptible to conversion to dopamine in the periphery, leading to side effects such as nausea, dyskinesias, and joint stiffness. To address this, inhibitors that reduce the breakdown of dopamine in the peripheral nervous system—called peripheral dopa decarboxylase inhibitors (carbidopa and benserazide) are given in combination with levodopa to reduce peripheral conversion that would otherwise devour most of the dose given. The addition of dopa decarbozylase inhibitors also maximizes bioavailabilty of dopamine in the brain, decreases side effects, and allows a lower dose of levodopa to be used.

Once in the brain, as dopamine travels from one cell to another, it can be broken down and rendered inactive by two enzymes, MAO (monoamine oxidase) and COMT (catechol-O-methyl transferase). One therapeutic strategy introduces a MAO inhibitor into the synapse, which interrupts the action of the MAO enzyme and prevents the breakdown of dopamine in the synapse. This allows more dopamine to remain in the synapse and increases the likelihood that it will bind to the postsynaptic membrane.

Although levodopa helps in at least three-quarters of parkinsonian cases, not all symptoms respond equally to the drug. Bradykinesia and rigidity respond best, while tremor may be only marginally reduced. Problems with balance and other symptoms may not be alleviated at all. Controlled release versions of levodopa in the form of intravenous and intestinal gel infusions spread out the medication and are showing promise.

Initial drug treatment may start with MAO-B inhibitors and dopamine agonists. Levodopa plus a dopa decarboxylase inhibitor (such as carbidopa) are used sparingly at first to delay as long as possible the side effects resulting from cumulative exposure of systemic dopaminergic function.

As the disease progresses and dopaminergic neurons continue to be lost in the substantia nigra, L-dopa eventually becomes ineffective for treating the motor symptoms and may concurrently cause dyskinesias. As medication becomes less effective, "off" periods may occur when the levodopa dose has worn off and movement is again difficult until a new dose is given. Medications to treat nonmovementrelated symptoms of PD, such as sleep disturbances and emotional problems, are also considered as needed.

After prolonged therapy with levodopa, a person with PD may alternate between phases with good response to medication and few symptoms (the "on" state) and phases with no response to medication and significant motor symptoms (the "off" state). Levodopa doses are therefore kept as low as possible, after using alternatives such as dopamine agonists and MAO-B inhibitors. Most people with PD will eventually require levodopa and hence later develop motor side effects such as involuntary movements (dyskinesia), painful leg cramps (dystonia), and a shortened response to each dose (motor fluctuations).

Prevention

Because the cause of Parkinson's is unknown, proven ways to prevent the disease also remain a mystery.

Some research has shown that regular aerobic exercise might reduce the risk of Parkinson's disease.

Some other research has shown that people who consume caffeine — which is found in coffee, tea and cola — get Parkinson's disease less often than those who don't drink it. Green tea is also related to a reduced risk of developing Parkinson's disease. However, it is still not known whether caffeine actually protects against getting Parkinson's, or is related in some other way. Currently there is not enough evidence to suggest drinking caffeinated beverages to protect against Parkinson's.

How is it managed and treated?

Exercise is recommended, as a treatment, to help manage depression for people with Parkinson's disease.

The following treatments may help people with Parkinson's disease manage depression:

antidepressant medication

exercise

counseling

A 2012 study found two types of antidepressants were effective in reducing the symptoms of depression in people with Parkinson's disease. These were:

selective serotonin reuptake inhibitors (SSRIs)

serotonin and norepinephrine reuptake inhibitors (SNRIs)

There are different brands of these antidepressant types available. A doctor can prescribe these. Also, the following strategies can help a person manage depression:

planning small goals that can be achieved each day

seeing friends and family, or speaking on the phone

trying to keep up leisure activities

reading about depression and trying to talk to close friends or family about it

Takeaway

It is common for a person diagnosed with Parkinson's disease to experience symptoms of depression.

Depression can have just as much of an impact on a person's life as the physical symptoms of Parkinson's disease. It is a psychological symptom of the condition that doctors believe is caused by changes in the brain's chemistry.

Fortunately, there are treatments available that may help people with Parkinson's disease manage depression. For this reason, it is crucial for a person with Parkinson's disease to discuss any symptoms of depression with their doctor.

The Role of Diet

Following a balanced diet improves general well-being and boosts your ability to deal with symptoms of the disease. Eating plenty of whole foods, such as fruits and vegetables, lean protein, beans and legumes, and whole grains, and staying hydrated are key ways to stay energized and healthy overall. That said, you should be aware of some special considerations.

- Constipation: Many patients with Parkinson's disease experience constipation due to a slowdown of the digestive system. At best, constipation is an annoyance, but at worst, your large intestine can become impacted. Combat constipation with a diet rich in fiber from sources such as fresh fruits and vegetables, whole grains, vegetables, legumes, and whole-grain breads and cereals. Drinking plenty of fluids and exercising can also help you avoid constipation.

- Dehydration: Medications that treat Parkinson's disease can dry you out. Not only can dehydration leave you more tired, over time, it can also lead to confusion, balance issues, weakness and kidney problems. Be sure to drink plenty of water and other fluids throughout the day.
- Medication interaction: The drug most commonly used to treat Parkinson's disease, carbidopa-levodopa, is absorbed in your small intestine. That absorption can be disrupted if you take your medication shortly after eating a high-protein meal, since it involves the same process. To help maximize the medication's effects, eat high-protein foods at other times of the day. If you take your medicine in the morning, have oatmeal rather than high-protein eggs for breakfast, and save your protein intake for later in the day.

When You Have No Appetite

Some days, you just may not feel like eating at all.

Talk to your doctor. Sometimes, depression can cause poor appetite. Your hunger likely will return when you get treatment.

Walk or do another light activity to rev up your appetite.

Drink beverages after you've finished eating so you don't feel full before the meal.

Include your favorite foods in your menu. Eat the high-calorie foods on your plate first. But avoid empty calories from sugary sodas, candies, and chips.

Perk up your meals by trying different dishes and ingredients.

Choose high-protein and high-calorie snacks, including:

- Ice cream

- Cheese

- Granola bars

- Custard

- Sandwiches

- Nachos with cheese

- Eggs

- Crackers with peanut butter

- Cereal with half and half

- Greek yogurt

Stay at a Healthy Weight

Malnutrition and weight loss are often problems for people with Parkinson's. So it's good to keep track of your weight.

Weigh yourself once or twice a week, unless your doctor says to do it more often. If you are taking diuretics or steroids, such as prednisone, you should step on the scale daily.

If you gain or lose weight noticeably (2 pounds in a day or 5 pounds in a week), talk to your doctor. They may want change your food and drinks to manage your condition.

If you need to gain weight:

Ask your doctor if nutritional supplements are right for you. Some can be harmful or interfere with your medication.

Avoid low-fat or low-calorie foods unless you've been told otherwise. Instead, use whole milk, whole milk cheese, and yogurt.

The Role of Exercise

Exercise can make the greatest impact on the course of your disease, says Denise Padilla-Davidson, a Johns Hopkins physical therapist who works with patients who have Parkinson's disease. "Movement, especially exercises that encourage balance and reciprocal patterns [movements that require coordination of both sides of your body], can actually slow progression of the disease," she says. Here's what you need to know:

Get your heart pumping: Many symptoms of Parkinson's disease that limit physical ability, such as impaired gait, problems with balance and strength, grip strength, and motor coordination, show improvement with regular cardiovascular exercise. For example, a review of studies on treadmill training found that regular walking workouts helped increase normal walking speed and lengthen stride length, which tends to shorten with Parkinson's disease.

Move it or lose it: As Parkinson's disease motor symptoms, like a slowed gait or tremor, become apparent, patients may become afraid of losing their balance and falling or dropping things, which leads to excessive caution and fear, which in turn leads to an even more sedentary lifestyle. Experts know that formal exercise helps keep patients active and healthy, and research also shows that normal physical activity may be just as or more important than trips to the gym. Keeping up with routine daily activities, like washing dishes, folding laundry, yardwork, shopping — anything that gets and keeps you on your feet — helps delay the degeneration of motor symptoms.

Work out your brain: Exercise — again, anything that gets your heart pumping — may help the brain maintain neuroplasticity, which is the ability to maintain old connections and form new ones between the neurons in your brain. "The neuroplasticity created from exercise in patients with Parkinson's disease may actually outweigh the effects of neurodegeneration," says Padilla-Davidson.

Recipes

Red Broccoli Salad

Recipe Summary

prep: 15 mins

cook: 35 mins

additional: 1 hr

total: 1 hr 50 mins

Servings: 11

Yield: 10 to 12 servings

Ingredients

- 2 pounds maple-flavored bacon
- 1 large head fresh broccoli, chopped
- ¾ cup chopped celery
- ¼ cup minced green onions
- ¼ cup diced red onion
- 1 ½ cups seedless grapes, halved
- ¾ cup blanched slivered almonds
- ¼ cup white sugar
- 2 tablespoons distilled white vinegar
- 1 cup mayonnaise

Directions

Instructions

Step 1

Place bacon in a large skillet. Cook, turning frequently, over medium high heat until evenly browned. Cool, and then crumble.

Step 2

Preheat oven to 300 degrees F (150 degrees C). Spread slivered almonds on a cookie sheet. Bake for approximately 12 to 14 minutes or until lightly browned, turning once during toasting. Cool.

Step 3

In a small bowl, mix together mayonnaise, sugar, and vinegar. Set aside.

Step 4

In a large bowl, combine broccoli, crumbled bacon, celery, green onions, red onions, grapes, and toasted almonds. Toss with mayonnaise dressing. Chill for several hours in the refrigerator.

Editor's Note:

The original submitter of this recipe, MAGGIE MCGUIRE, has let us know that 1 pound bacon is all you need for this recipe, and that 2 pounds might be too much.

Nutrition Facts

Per Serving:

382 calories; protein 12.9g; carbohydrates 13.7g; fat 31.2g; cholesterol 37.5mg; sodium 759.9mg.

Shredded Apple Carrot Salad

Recipe Summary

prep: 15 mins

cook: 5 mins

total: 20 mins

Servings: 6

Yield: 6 servings

Ingredients

2 tablespoons sesame seeds

2 cups shredded carrots

1 Granny Smith apple, cored and shredded

½ cup chopped fresh parsley

¼ cup lemon juice

2 tablespoons apple cider vinegar

1 tablespoon white sugar (Optional)

1 clove garlic, minced

1 teaspoon salt

½ teaspoon ground black pepper

2 tablespoons safflower oil

Directions

Instructions

Step 1

Heat a skillet over medium heat; pour sesame seeds into the hot skillet. Cook, stirring often, until sesame seeds are lightly browned and fragrant, 3 to 5 minutes. Remove from heat.

Step 2

Mix carrots, apple, toasted sesame seeds, and parsley together in a bowl.

Step 3

Whisk lemon juice, vinegar, sugar, garlic, salt, and pepper together in a separate bowl; slowly drizzle safflower oil into lemon juice mixture while continuing to whisk. Pour dressing over carrot mixture; toss to coat.

Cook's Note:

Substitute honey or maple syrup for the sugar, if desired.

Nutrition Facts

Per Serving:

97 calories; protein 1.2g; carbohydrates 10.7g; fat 6.2g; sodium 416.8mg.

Fresh Broccoli Salad

Recipe Summary

prep: 15 mins

cook: 15 mins

total: 30 mins

Servings: 9

Yield: 8 to 10 servings

Ingredients

  2 heads fresh broccoli

  1 red onion

  ½ pound bacon

  ¾ cup raisins

  ¾ cup sliced almonds

1 cup mayonnaise

½ cup white sugar

2 tablespoons white wine vinegar

Directions

Instructions

Step 1

Place bacon in a deep skillet and cook over medium high heat until evenly brown. Cool and crumble.

Step 2

Cut the broccoli into bite-size pieces and cut the onion into thin bite-size slices. Combine with the bacon, raisins, your favorite nuts and mix well.

Step 3

To prepare the dressing, mix the mayonnaise, sugar and vinegar together until smooth. Stir into the salad, let chill and serve.

Nutrition Facts

Per Serving:

374 calories; protein 7.3g; carbohydrates 28.5g; fat 27.2g; cholesterol 18.3mg; sodium 352.9mg.

Recipe Summary

prep: 15 mins

additional: 1 hr

total: 1 hr 15 mins

Servings: 12

Yield: 12 servings

Ingredients

- 4 cups shredded carrots

- 4 cups chopped apples

- 1 cup creamy salad dressing (such as Miracle Whip®)

- 1 cup raisins

- 1 cup chopped pecans

Directions

Instructions

Step 1

Lightly mix carrots, apples, creamy salad dressing, raisins, and pecans in a large bowl.

Step 2

Chill completely, about 1 hour.

Nutrition Facts

Per Serving:

198 calories; protein 1.7g; carbohydrates 23.3g; fat 12.1g; cholesterol 6.7mg; sodium 197.9mg.

Alyson's Broccoli Salad

Recipe Summary

prep: 15 mins

cook: 15 mins

total: 30 mins

Servings: 6

Yield: 6 servings

Ingredients

10 slices bacon

1 head fresh broccoli, cut into bite size pieces

¼ cup red onion, chopped

½ cup raisins

3 tablespoons white wine vinegar

2 tablespoons white sugar

1 cup mayonnaise

1 cup sunflower seeds

Directions

Instructions

Step 1

Place bacon in a large, deep skillet. Cook over medium high heat until evenly brown. Drain, crumble and set aside.

Step 2

In a medium bowl, combine the broccoli, onion and raisins. In a small bowl, whisk together the vinegar, sugar and mayonnaise. Pour over broccoli mixture, and toss until well mixed. Refrigerate for at least two hours.

Step 3

Before serving, toss salad with crumbled bacon and sunflower seeds.

Nutrition Facts

Per Serving:

559 calories; protein 12.9g; carbohydrates 23.9g; fat 48.1g; cholesterol 30.8mg; sodium 583.5mg.

Recipe Summary

prep: 10 mins

cook: 1 hr

additional: 5 mins

total: 1 hr 15 mins

Servings: 6

Yield: 6 servings

Ingredients

  2 tablespoons olive oil

  1 onion, chopped

  1 small carrot, chopped

  1 stalk celery, chopped

  1 pinch salt

  1 cup pearl barley

  1 ½ cups chicken stock

  ¾ cup water

  2 teaspoons dried thyme

  2 teaspoons dried sage

5 large fresh mint leaves, chopped, or more to taste

Directions

Instructions

Step 1

Heat olive oil in a heavy-bottomed pot over medium heat; cook and stir onion until translucent, about 5 minutes. Add carrot, celery, and salt; cook and stir for 2 minutes. Add barley and mix to coat with oil; cook and stir until barley is golden brown, about 5 minutes.

Step 2

Stir chicken stock, water, thyme, and sage into barley mixture. Cover pot and bring to a boil; reduce heat to medium-low and simmer until liquid is absorbed, about 45 minutes. Remove pot from heat and stir mint into barley pilaf. Cover pot and allow flavors to blend, 5 to 10 minutes.

Cook's Note:

Additional salt may be needed if low sodium broth is used.

Nutrition Facts

Per Serving:

174 calories; protein 3.8g; carbohydrates 29.3g; fat 5.2g; cholesterol 0.2mg; sodium 213.3mg.

Recipe Summary

prep: 15 mins

cook: 15 mins

additional: 1 hr

total: 1 hr 30 mins

Servings: 10

Yield: 10 servings

Ingredients

- 2 (9 ounce) packages refrigerated three-cheese tortellini
- 1 pound bacon
- 4 cups chopped broccoli
- 1 pint grape tomatoes, halved
- 2 green onions, finely chopped
- 1 cup bottled coleslaw dressing

Directions

Instructions

Step 1

Cook the tortellini according to the package directions, drain, rinse with cold water, and refrigerate until cool, about 30 minutes.

Step 2

Place the bacon in a large, deep skillet, and cook over medium-high heat, turning occasionally, until evenly browned, about 10 minutes. Drain the bacon slices on a paper towel-lined plate. Chop the bacon into 1/2-inch pieces while still a little warm.

Step 3

Place the tortellini, bacon, broccoli, grape tomatoes, and green onions into a salad bowl. Pour the dressing over the ingredients, and toss lightly to coat. Chill in refrigerator before serving.

Cook's Notes

You can use whole wheat three cheese tortellini, which can usually be found in the refrigerated section of the store, low sodium bacon or turkey bacon, and light coleslaw dressing.

I suggest starting to cook the tortellini before you start chopping your veggies, since it takes the longest to cool, and then placing it in the refrigerator until you are done with everything else.

Nutrition Facts

Per Serving:

349 calories; protein 13.9g; carbohydrates 33.6g; fat 18.2g; cholesterol 46.9mg; sodium 736.1mg.

Apple Coffee Cake

Recipe Summary

prep: 20 mins

cook: 35 mins

total: 55 mins

Servings: 8

Yield: 1 8-inch square cake

Ingredients

cooking spray

1 tablespoon flour, or as needed

Cake:

¼ cup butter, softened

¾ cup brown sugar

1 large egg

¼ cup sour cream

¼ cup vanilla yogurt

1 teaspoon vanilla extract

1 cup all-purpose flour

¾ teaspoon ground cinnamon

½ teaspoon baking soda

¼ teaspoon salt

2 cups diced Granny Smith apple

Topping:

¼ cup brown sugar

¼ cup all-purpose flour

2 tablespoons butter

½ teaspoon ground cinnamon

Directions

Instructions

Step 1

Preheat oven to 350 degrees F (175 degrees C). Spray an 8-inch square baking dish with cooking spray; dust with 1 tablespoon flour.

Step 2

Beat 1/4 cup butter and 3/4 cup brown sugar together with an electric mixer in a large bowl until light and fluffy. The mixture should be noticeably lighter in color. Beat egg into butter mixture. Add sour cream, vanilla yogurt, and vanilla extract to the mixture; beat to integrate.

Step 3

Stir 1 cup flour, 3/4 teaspoon cinnamon, baking soda, and salt together in a bowl; add to the butter mixture and beat to combine into a batter. Fold apples into the batter. Pour batter into prepared baking dish.

Step 4

Mix 1/4 cup brown sugar, 1/4 cup flour, 2 tablespoons butter, and 1/2 teaspoon cinnamon together in a bowl using a fork to achieve a crumbly consistency; sprinkle over the top of the batter.

Step 5

Bake in the preheated oven until a toothpick inserted into the center comes out clean, 35 to 40 minutes. Cool in the pan for 10 minutes before removing to cool completely on a wire rack.

Cook's Note:

If you don't have vanilla yogurt on hand, add 1/4 cup more sour cream or Greek yogurt to the recipe with a dash more vanilla. I like to serve each piece with a dollop of vanilla yogurt on top!

Nutrition Facts

Per Serving:

275 calories; protein 3.6g; carbohydrates 41.4g; fat 11g; cholesterol 46.9mg; sodium 235.7mg.

Tex-Mex Pasta Salad

Recipe Summary

prep: 15 mins

cook: 20 mins

additional: 1 hr

total: 1 hr 35 mins

Servings: 10

Yield: 10 servings

Ingredients

- 2 tablespoons olive oil

- 1 teaspoon salt

- 1 (16 ounce) package fusilli pasta

- 2 pounds extra lean ground beef

- 1 (1.25 ounce) package taco seasoning mix

1 (24 ounce) jar mild salsa

1 (8 ounce) bottle ranch dressing

1 ½ red bell peppers, chopped

6 green onions, chopped

¾ cup chopped pickled jalapeno peppers

1 (2.25 ounce) can sliced black olives (Optional)

1 (8 ounce) package shredded Cheddar cheese

Directions

Instructions

Step 1

Fill a large pot with water; pour in the olive oil and salt. Bring to a rolling boil over high heat. Stir in the fusilli, and return to a boil. Cook the pasta uncovered, stirring occasionally, until the pasta has cooked through, but is still firm to the bite, about 9 minutes. Drain and set aside.

Step 2

Heat a large skillet over medium-high heat and stir in the ground beef. Cook and stir until the beef is crumbly, evenly browned, and no longer pink. Drain and discard any excess grease. Mix in taco seasoning mix, remove from heat, and cool completely.

Step 3

Combine salsa, ranch dressing, bell peppers, green onions, jalapenos, and black olives in a medium bowl. Toss together the cooked pasta, cooled beef mixture, Cheddar cheese, and dressing mixture in a large bowl. Cover and refrigerate at least 1 hour before serving.

Nutrition Facts

Per Serving:

597 calories; protein 29.9g; carbohydrates 43.2g; fat 34g; cholesterol 84.9mg; sodium 1540.9mg.

Sesame Chicken Pasta Salad

Recipe Summary

prep: 20 mins

cook: 10 mins

total: 30 mins

Servings: 6

Yield: 6 servings

Ingredients

  1 (12 ounce) package radiatore pasta

  ¼ cup sesame seeds

  ¼ cup salad oil

  ¾ cup soy sauce

½ cup white wine vinegar

3 ½ tablespoons sugar

2 cups cubed, cooked chicken

½ cup chopped fresh parsley

½ cup coarsely chopped green onion

4 cups torn fresh spinach leaves

Directions

Instructions

Step 1

Bring a large pot of lightly salted water to a boil. Add pasta and cook for 8 to 10 minutes or until al dente; drain.

Step 2

Meanwhile, heat oil in a small skillet over medium-low heat. Stir in sesame seeds and cook until golden brown. Remove from heat. Stir in soy sauce, vinegar, and sugar. Pour dressing into a sealable container, and set aside.

Step 3

In a large bowl, mix together pasta, cooked chicken, and 1 cup dressing (reserve remaining dressing). Cover salad, and refrigerate at least 6 hours.

Step 4

Directly before serving, stir in parsley, green onions, and spinach. Toss with remaining dressing, if desired.

Nutrition Facts

Per Serving:

475 calories; protein 23.3g; carbohydrates 54g; fat 19.4g; cholesterol 36.4mg; sodium 1871.2mg.

Blueberry, Banana, and Peanut Butter Smoothie

Recipe Summary

prep: 10 mins

total: 10 mins

Servings: 2

Yield: 2 cups

Ingredients

1 tablespoon flax seed meal or wheat germ

1 banana

½ cup frozen blueberries

1 tablespoon peanut butter

1 teaspoon honey

½ cup plain yogurt

1 cup milk

Directions

Instructions

Step 1

Put ground flax seed meal or wheat germ into blender to grind and further breakdown. This will also eliminate any bitterness from the flax seed.

Step 2

Place the banana, blueberries, peanut butter, honey, yogurt, and milk into the blender. Cover, and puree until smooth. Pour into glasses to serve.

Nutrition Facts

Per Serving:

251 calories; protein 10.8g; carbohydrates 34.4g; fat 9.2g; cholesterol 13.4mg; sodium 132.4mg.

Marinated Beet Salad

Recipe Summary

prep: 10 mins

cook: 10 mins

additional: 4 hrs

total: 4 hrs 20 mins

Servings: 4

Yield: 4 servings

Ingredients

1 (16 ounce) can whole beets

¼ cup white sugar

1 teaspoon prepared mustard

¼ cup white wine vinegar

¼ cup diced red onion

Directions

Instructions

Step 1

Drain beets, reserving 1/4 cup liquid, and slice into 1/4 to 1/2 inch slivers. Add onions and toss.

Step 2

In a saucepan over medium heat, cook the sugar, mustard and reserved 1/4 cup liquid until dissolved. Add vinegar and bring to boil; remove from heat and allow to cool.

Step 3

Pour over the beet slices and onions, toss and refrigerate for 4 to 6 hours. Remove from refrigerator and serve at room temperature.

Nutrition Facts

Per Serving:

89 calories; protein 1.2g; carbohydrates 21.7g; fat 0.2g; sodium 236.3mg.

Broccoli Beet Salad with Raspberry Vinaigrette
Recipe Summary

prep: 20 mins

total: 20 mins

Servings: 8

Yield: 8 servings

Ingredients

2 heads broccoli, cut into bite-size pieces

½ red onion, cut into slivers

1 (15 ounce) can dark red kidney beans, rinsed and drained

1 (14.5 ounce) can no-salt-added beets - drained, rinsed, and halved

⅓ cup raspberry jam

½ cup red wine vinegar

¼ cup olive oil

¼ teaspoon salt

1 cup pecans

¼ cup crumbled goat cheese

Directions

Instructions

Step 1

Mix broccoli, red onion, kidney beans, and beets in a large bowl.

Step 2

Whisk raspberry jam, vinegar, olive oil, and salt in a small bowl; pour over vegetable mixture. Toss broccoli salad with pecans and goat cheese.

Nutrition Facts

Per Serving:

296 calories; protein 7.6g; carbohydrates 29.2g; fat 18.4g; cholesterol 3.5mg; sodium 243.9mg.

Recipe Summary

prep: 20 mins

cook: 30 mins

total: 50 mins

Servings: 6

Yield: 6 servings

Ingredients

6 tablespoons vegetable oil

2 cloves garlic, chopped

6 tablespoons soy sauce

6 tablespoons rice vinegar

1 tablespoon Thai chili sauce

3 tablespoons honey

8 ounces extra-firm tofu, cut into 1/4-inch cubes

½ (16 ounce) package linguine pasta

1 tablespoon sesame oil

8 ounces bean sprouts

8 ounces shredded carrots

1 green bell pepper, thinly sliced

8 green onions, halved lengthwise

Directions

Instructions

Step 1

Heat the vegetable oil in a wok over medium-high heat; cook and stir the garlic until lightly browned, about 2 minutes. Pour in the soy sauce, rice vinegar, chili sauce, and honey, stir to mix, and bring the mixture to a simmer. Reduce heat to medium-low, and let the sauce simmer for 10 minutes. Transfer the sauce to a bowl, and stir the tofu into the sauce. Set the tofu mixture aside.

Step 2

Fill a large pot with lightly salted water and bring to a rolling boil over high heat. Once the water is boiling, stir in the linguine, and return to a boil. Cook the pasta uncovered, stirring occasionally, until the pasta has cooked through, but is still firm to the bite, about 11 minutes. Drain well in a colander set in the sink.

Step 3

While the pasta is boiling, heat the sesame oil in clean wok or large skillet; cook and stir the bean sprouts, carrots, green pepper, and green onions until the vegetables are bright in color and slightly wilted, about 5 minutes. Pour in the tofu with sauce and linguine; stir to combine.

Nutrition Facts

Per Serving:

388 calories; protein 11.8g; carbohydrates 46.6g; fat 19.2g; sodium 1045mg.

Pumpkin and Tofu Miso Soup

Recipe Summary

prep: 15 mins

cook: 15 mins

total: 30 mins

Servings: 2

Yield: 2 servings

Ingredients

¼ small pumpkin - peeled, seeded, and cubed

1 (2 inch) piece fresh ginger, cut into matchsticks

2 tablespoons soy sauce

2 ounces buckwheat noodles

3 ½ ounces firm tofu, cubed

2 teaspoons miso paste

2 teaspoons sesame oil

2 green onions, finely chopped on the diagonal

2 large red chile peppers, sliced on the diagonal

2 tablespoons toasted sesame seeds

2 tablespoons chopped fresh cilantro, or more to taste

2 tablespoons pickled ginger

Directions

Instructions

Step 1

Bring a large saucepan of water to a boil; add pumpkin, ginger, and soy sauce. Cook pumpkin mixture for about 3 minutes. Add noodles to pumpkin mixture and cook until noodles are slightly cooked, about 4 minutes.

Step 2

Stir tofu into pumpkin-noodle mixture and cook until pumpkin and noodles are almost tender, 5 to 10 more minutes.

Step 3

Place 1 teaspoon miso paste into each serving bowl. Ladle cooking water into each bowl and whisk until miso is dissolved.

Step 4

Divide pumpkin-tofu soup between the 2 serving bowls; garnish each with 1 teaspoon sesame oil, 1 chopped green onion, 1 sliced red chile pepper, 1 tablespoon sesame seeds, 1 tablespoon cilantro, and 1 tablespoon pickled ginger.

Nutrition Facts

Per Serving:

317 calories; protein 12g; carbohydrates 40.9g; fat 12.8g; sodium 1230.8mg.

Cranberry Pumpkin Muffins

Recipe Summary

prep: 20 mins

cook: 20 mins

total: 40 mins

Servings: 12

Yield: 12 servings

Ingredients

- 2 cups all-purpose flour
- ¾ cup brown sugar, packed
- 2 teaspoons baking powder
- ¼ teaspoon baking soda
- ½ teaspoon salt
- 1 teaspoon ground cinnamon
- ¼ teaspoon ground ginger
- ⅛ teaspoon ground cloves
- ⅛ teaspoon ground nutmeg
- 1 cup canned unsweetened pumpkin puree
- 2 eggs, lightly beaten
- ½ cup butter, melted
- ¼ cup buttermilk
- 2 teaspoons vanilla extract
- 1 cup dried, sweetened cranberries

Directions

Instructions

Step 1

Preheat oven to 400 degrees F (200 degrees C). Grease or place paper muffin cups in a 12 cup muffin tin.

Step 2

Mix the flour, brown sugar, baking powder, baking soda, salt, cinnamon, ginger, cloves, and nutmeg together in a mixing bowl.

Step 3

Beat the canned pumpkin, eggs, butter, buttermilk, and vanilla together in another large mixing bowl. Gradually beat in the flour mixture until well blended. Stir in the dried cranberries until evenly blended. Spoon batter into muffin tins about 3/4 full.

Step 4

Bake in preheated oven until a toothpick inserted in the middle of a muffin comes out clean, 20 to 25 minutes. 3 minutes before turning out from pan. Serve warm or at room temperature.

Nutrition Facts

Per Serving:

253 calories; protein 3.7g; carbohydrates 40.2g; fat 8.8g; cholesterol 51.5mg; sodium 329.5mg

Lime Chicken and Mushroom Pasta

Recipe Summary

prep: 25 mins

cook: 15 mins

total: 40 mins

Servings: 6

Yield: 6 servings

Ingredients

- 4 tablespoons olive oil

- 2 limes, juiced

- 4 skinless, boneless chicken breast halves - cut into 1 inch cubes

- 1 pound fresh mushrooms, quartered

- 1 red bell pepper, thinly sliced

- 1 yellow bell pepper, thinly sliced

- 1 cup chopped fresh cilantro

- 1 (16 ounce) package linguini pasta

Directions

Instructions

Step 1

Cook pasta in a large pot of boiling salted water until al dente.

Step 2

Heat a large, non-stick skillet over medium high heat. Add olive oil and chicken, and saute slightly. Add mushrooms and peppers; saute until peppers are soft but crisp. Stir in lime juice and cilantro.

Step 3

Drain pasta, and transfer to a large serving bowl. Top with chicken mixture, and toss slightly. Garnish with lime slices.

Nutrition Facts

Per Serving:

466 calories; protein 28.4g; carbohydrates 62.6g; fat 12.8g; cholesterol 40.6mg; sodium 46.4mg..

Fresh Tomato Sauce

Recipe Summary

prep: 5 mins

cook: 30 mins

total: 35 mins

Servings: 6

Yield: 6 servings

Ingredients

¼ cup olive oil

6 tomatoes, chopped

3 onions, minced

2 green bell peppers, minced

4 cloves garlic, minced

3 tablespoons white wine

salt and pepper to taste

Directions

Instructions

Step 1

In a large saucepan, heat oil over medium heat; add tomatoes, onions, green bell peppers, garlic, white wine and salt and pepper to taste.

Step 2

Mix ingredients well; cover and simmer for 30 minutes. Serve.

Nutrition Facts

Per Serving:

144 calories; protein 2.2g; carbohydrates 13.4g; fat 9.4g; sodium 10.1mg.

Recipe Summary

prep: 5 mins

cook: 10 mins

additional: 23 hrs 20 mins

total: 23 hrs 35 mins

Servings: 8

Yield: 8 servings

Ingredients

   1 (15 ounce) can peas, drained

   1 (15 ounce) can shoe peg corn, drained

   1 (15 ounce) can green beans, drained

   1 (2 ounce) jar pimentos

   1 cup chopped celery

½ cup chopped green bell pepper

½ cup chopped onion

1 cup white sugar

½ teaspoon ground black pepper

1 teaspoon salt

½ cup vegetable oil

¾ cup white wine vinegar

Directions

Instructions

Step 1

Mix together the peas, corn, green beans, pimentos, celery, bell pepper and onion.

Step 2

In a saucepan over medium heat, combine the sugar, black pepper, salt, oil and vinegar. Bring to a boil and pour over salad; mix well to coat. Refrigerate for 24 hours.

Nutrition Facts

Per Serving:

307 calories; protein 4g; carbohydrates 43.7g; fat 14.5g; sodium 723.7mg.

Recipe Summary

prep: 10 mins

cook: 10 mins

additional: 4 hrs

total: 4 hrs 20 mins

Servings: 4

Yield: 4 servings

Ingredients

1 (16 ounce) can whole beets

¼ cup white sugar

1 teaspoon prepared mustard

¼ cup white wine vinegar

¼ cup diced red onion

Directions

Instructions

Step 1

Drain beets, reserving 1/4 cup liquid, and slice into 1/4 to 1/2 inch slivers. Add onions and toss.

Step 2

In a saucepan over medium heat, cook the sugar, mustard and reserved 1/4 cup liquid until dissolved. Add vinegar and bring to boil; remove from heat and allow to cool.

Step 3

Pour over the beet slices and onions, toss and refrigerate for 4 to 6 hours. Remove from refrigerator and serve at room temperature.

Nutrition Facts

Per Serving:

89 calories; protein 1.2g; carbohydrates 21.7g; fat 0.2g; sodium 236.3mg.

Mushroom Barley Soup

Recipe Summary

prep: 25 mins

cook: 40 mins

total: 1 hr 5 mins

Servings: 6

Yield: 6 servings

Ingredients

1 cup barley

3 cups water

1 ½ tablespoons olive oil

2 onions, chopped

1 carrot, thinly sliced

2 stalks celery, thinly sliced

2 (10 ounce) packages sliced mushrooms

5 cups beef broth

½ teaspoon salt

¼ teaspoon ground black pepper

Directions

Instructions

Step 1

Bring the barley and water to a boil in a saucepan. Cover, reduce heat to low, and simmer 30 minutes, or until tender.

Step 2

Meanwhile, heat olive oil in a large saucepan over medium heat, stir in the onions, carrots, and celery; cook and stir until the onion has softened and turned translucent, about 10 minutes. Stir in mushrooms, and cook 5 minutes more.

Step 3

Pour in beef broth, and bring soup to a simmer over medium-high heat, then reduce heat to medium-low, and continue simmering 15 minutes. Stir in barley, and season with salt and pepper before serving.

Nutrition Facts

Per Serving:

194 calories; protein 9.6g; carbohydrates 30.5g; fat 4.9g; sodium 882.4mg.

Summer Fresh Shrimp Kebabs

Recipe Summary

prep: 15 mins

cook: 5 mins

additional: 1 hr

total: 1 hr 20 mins

Servings: 4

Yield: 8 kebabs

Ingredients

- 1 bunch fresh cilantro, chopped
- ½ bunch fresh parsley, chopped
- 3 cloves garlic, finely chopped
- 1 shallot, finely chopped
- 2 lemons, zested and juiced
- 1 lime, zested and juiced
- ¼ cup extra-virgin olive oil
- 40 extra-large shrimp, peeled and deveined
- 8 skewers

Directions

Instructions

Step 1

Combine cilantro, parsley, garlic, shallot, lemon zest and juice, and lime zest and juice in a small bowl. Whisk in olive oil slowly until marinade is combined.

Step 2

Place shrimp in a large zip-top bag and pour in marinade mixture. Seal bag and gently massage onto shrimp. Refrigerate for 1 to 6 hours.

Step 3

Preheat an outdoor grill for medium-high heat and lightly oil the grate. Slide 5 shrimp onto each skewer.

Step 4

Grill shrimp kebabs until they are bright pink on the outside and meat is opaque, about 2 minutes per side. Serve hot.

Nutrition Facts

Per Serving:

380 calories; protein 48g; carbohydrates 11.6g; fat 16.7g; cholesterol 431.4mg; sodium 510.1mg.

Red Beans and Rice

Recipe Summary

prep: 15 mins

cook: 30 mins

total: 45 mins

Servings: 5

Yield: 4 to 6 servings

Ingredients

1 (14 ounce) package boil in bag rice

1 ½ pounds lean ground beef

2 (15 ounce) cans kidney beans, drained and rinsed

1 (24 ounce) jar picante sauce

1 ½ tablespoons paprika

1 tablespoon chili powder

½ teaspoon crushed red pepper flakes

12 ounces shredded sharp Cheddar cheese

Directions

Instructions

Step 1

Cook the rice according to package directions.

Step 2

Place the ground beef in a large skillet over medium high heat. Saute for 5 to 10 minutes, or until browned and crumbly. Drain well and transfer meat to a large pot over low heat. Add the rice, beans, picante sauce, paprika, chili powder and crushed red pepper flakes. Stir well and let simmer for 20 minutes. Stir in cheese and let simmer for 10 more minutes.

Nutrition Facts

Per Serving:

1123 calories; protein 58.5g; carbohydrates 99.9g; fat 52.4g; cholesterol 173.6mg; sodium 1573.7mg.

Picnic Potato Salad with No Mayonnaise

Recipe Summary

prep: 15 mins

cook: 10 mins

additional: 30 mins

total: 55 mins

Servings: 6

Yield: 6 servings

Ingredients

2 pounds small new potatoes, quartered

2 tablespoons balsamic vinegar

¼ cup extra-virgin olive oil

1 tablespoon Dijon mustard

2 tablespoons chopped fresh basil

½ teaspoon salt

¼ teaspoon ground black pepper

½ cup chopped onion

¾ cup crumbled blue cheese

2 tablespoons chopped fresh chives

Directions

Instructions

Step 1

Place potatoes into a large pot and cover with lightly salted water; bring to a boil. Reduce heat to medium-low and simmer until tender, 10 to 15 minutes; drain.

Step 2

Whisk vinegar, olive oil, mustard, basil, salt, and pepper together in a large bowl; add the potatoes and onion. Toss gently to coat. Let stand until cool, about 30 minutes.

Step 3

Fold blue cheese and chives into potato salad until blended.

Editor's Note:

Picnic salads, with or without mayonnaise, should be kept refrigerated or in a cooler. For food safety reasons, always refrigerate potato salads after 2 hours at room temperature, or 1 hour on hot days--at or above 90 degrees F (32 degrees C).

Nutrition Facts

Per Serving:

272 calories; protein 6.9g; carbohydrates 29.5g; fat 14.4g; cholesterol 12.7mg; sodium 502.7mg.

Stuffed Peppers

Recipe Summary

prep: 20 mins

cook: 1 hr

total: 1 hr 20 mins

Servings: 6

Yield: 6 servings

Ingredients

1 pound ground beef

½ cup uncooked long grain white rice

1 cup water

6 green bell peppers

2 (8 ounce) cans tomato sauce

1 tablespoon Worcestershire sauce

¼ teaspoon garlic powder

¼ teaspoon onion powder

salt and pepper to taste

1 teaspoon Italian seasoning

Directions

Instructions

Step 1

Preheat oven to 350 degrees F (175 degrees C).

Step 2

Place the rice and water in a saucepan, and bring to a boil. Reduce heat, cover, and cook 20 minutes. In a skillet over medium heat, cook the beef until evenly browned.

Step 3

Remove and discard the tops, seeds, and membranes of the bell peppers. Arrange peppers in a baking dish with the hollowed sides facing upward. (Slice the bottoms of the peppers if necessary so that they will stand upright.)

Step 4

In a bowl, mix the browned beef, cooked rice, 1 can tomato sauce, Worcestershire sauce, garlic powder, onion powder, salt, and pepper. Spoon an equal amount of the mixture into each hollowed pepper. Mix the remaining tomato sauce and Italian seasoning in a bowl, and pour over the stuffed peppers.

Step 5

Bake 1 hour in the preheated oven, basting with sauce every 15 minutes, until the peppers are tender.

Nutrition Facts

Per Serving:

248 calories; protein 16g; carbohydrates 25.6g; fat 9.4g; cholesterol 45.9mg; sodium 563.6mg.

Strawberry Cream Cheese Spread

Recipe Summary

prep: 5 mins

total: 5 mins

Servings: 8

Yield: 8 servings

Ingredients

- 1 (8 ounce) package cream cheese, softened

- 2 tablespoons confectioners' sugar

- 1 cup fresh strawberries, hulled

Directions

Instructions

Step 1

In a blender or food processor, combine the cream cheese, confectioners' sugar, and strawberries. Pulse until smooth and well blended. Use immediately, or refrigerate until needed.

Nutrition Facts

Per Serving:

112 calories; protein 2.2g; carbohydrates 4.2g; fat 9.8g; cholesterol 30.8mg; sodium 83.1mg.

Stuffed Cabbage Soup

Recipe Summary

prep: 10 mins

cook: 1 hr

total: 1 hr 10 mins

Servings: 8

Yield: 8 servings

Ingredients

- 1 tablespoon vegetable oil

- 1 pound ground beef

- 1 (14 ounce) package classic coleslaw mix

- 1 large onion, chopped

- 2 (14 ounce) cans beef broth

- 1 (28 ounce) can crushed tomatoes in puree

- 1 cup water

- ½ cup light brown sugar

- 1 tablespoon fresh lemon juice

- 1 teaspoon salt

- ⅓ cup long-grain rice

Directions

Instructions

Step 1

Heat oil in a large pot over medium-high heat. Cook and stir ground beef in the hot skillet until browned and crumbly, 5 to 7 minutes. Add coleslaw mix and onion; cook for 4 minutes. Add broth, tomatoes, water, brown sugar, lemon juice, and salt.

Step 2

Bring mixture to a boil, add rice, and reduce heat to medium-low. Cover and let simmer until rice is tender, about 45 minutes.

Cook's Notes:

You can use ground turkey instead of beef, if preferred. If you don't want to use bagged cabbage, shred a small cabbage instead.

Nutrition Facts

Per Serving:

283 calories; protein 13.7g; carbohydrates 35g; fat 10.4g; cholesterol 39.4mg; sodium 793.6mg.

Recipe Summary

prep: 15 mins

cook: 40 mins

total: 55 mins

Servings: 12

Yield: 12 servings

Ingredients

- 1 small butternut squash, cubed

- 2 red bell peppers, seeded and diced

- 1 sweet potato, peeled and cubed

- 3 Yukon Gold potatoes, cubed

- 1 red onion, quartered

- 1 tablespoon chopped fresh thyme

- 2 tablespoons chopped fresh rosemary

- ¼ cup olive oil

- 2 tablespoons balsamic vinegar

- salt and freshly ground black pepper

Directions

Instructions

Step 1

Preheat oven to 475 degrees F (245 degrees C).

Step 2

In a large bowl, combine the squash, red bell peppers, sweet potato, and Yukon Gold potatoes. Separate the red onion quarters into pieces, and add them to the mixture.

Step 3

In a small bowl, stir together thyme, rosemary, olive oil, vinegar, salt, and pepper. Toss with vegetables until they are coated. Spread evenly on a large roasting pan.

Step 4

Roast for 35 to 40 minutes in the preheated oven, stirring every 10 minutes, or until vegetables are cooked through and browned.

Nutrition Facts

Per Serving:

123 calories; protein 2g; carbohydrates 20g; fat 4.7g; sodium 26mg.

Recipe Summary

prep: 20 mins

cook: 40 mins

total: 1 hr

Servings: 8

Yield: 8 cabbage rolls

Ingredients

⅔ cup water

⅓ cup uncooked white rice

8 cabbage leaves

1 pound lean ground beef

¼ cup chopped onion

1 egg, slightly beaten

1 teaspoon salt

¼ teaspoon ground black pepper

1 (10.75 ounce) can condensed tomato soup

Directions

Instructions

Step 1

In a medium saucepan, bring water to a boil. Add rice and stir. Reduce heat, cover and simmer for 20 minutes.

Step 2

Bring a large, wide saucepan of lightly salted water to a boil. Add cabbage leaves and cook for 2 to 4 minutes or until softened; drain.

Step 3

In a medium mixing bowl, combine the ground beef, 1 cup cooked rice, onion, egg, salt and pepper, along with 2 tablespoons of tomato soup. Mix thoroughly.

Step 4

Divide the beef mixture evenly among the cabbage leaves. Roll and secure them with toothpicks or string.

Step 5

In a large skillet over medium heat, place the cabbage rolls and pour the remaining tomato soup over the top. Cover and bring to a boil. Reduce heat to low and simmer for about 40 minutes, stirring and basting with the liquid often.

Nutrition Facts

Per Serving:

223 calories; protein 12.8g; carbohydrates 13.3g; fat 13.1g; cholesterol 65.8mg; sodium 656.9mg.